T0144617

THE ACID DANGER

COMBATING ACIDOSIS CORRECTLY

DR. WOLFGANG R. AUER

Basic
Health
PUBLICATIONS, INC.

The information contained in this book is based upon the research and personal and professional experiences of the author. It is not intended as a substitute for consulting with your physician or other healthcare provider. Any attempt to diagnose and treat an illness should be done under the direction of a healthcare professional.

The publisher does not advocate the use of any particular healthcare protocol but believes the information in this book should be available to the public. The publisher and author are not responsible for any adverse effects or consequences resulting from the use of the suggestions, preparations, or procedures discussed in this book. Should the reader have any questions concerning the appropriateness of any procedures or preparation mentioned, the author and the publisher strongly suggest consulting a professional healthcare advisor.

Basic Health Publications, Inc.
www.basichealthpub.com

Library of Congress Cataloging-in-Publication Data

Auer, Wolfgang R.

  The acid danger : combating acidosis correctly / Wolfgang R. Auer.
    p. cm.
  Includes bibliographical references and index.
  ISBN: 978-1-59120-080-2 (Pbk.)
  ISBN: 978-1-68162-788-5 (Hardcover)
  1. Acidosis—Popular works. I. Title.

  RC630.A93   2004
  616.3'992—dc22

                       2004017091

Editors: Carol Rosenberg/Karen Anspach
Typesetter: Gary A. Rosenberg
Cover Designer: Mike Stromberg

Contents

Introduction

Acidosis is a condition in which the acid/alkaline balance (more familiarly known as the pH balance) of the body has shifted unfavorably and body fluids have become excessively acidic. While many people are acquainted with the concept of acidosis, or a negative shift in pH balance, most are unaware of its relationship to other diseases or health problems. Acidosis is often at the root of many common health complaints, but it usually isn't considered a cause of disease until after a health problem has been wrongly diagnosed and unsuccessfully treated for years. This is unfortunate. All too often, acidosis-related health problems are not recognized as such and are diagnosed as incurable and treated improperly. Many people are led to believe that they have no choice but to learn to live with the assorted complications of acidosis without knowing exactly what they're up against.

Fortunately, numerous people with acidosis-related conditions have benefited from undergoing a deacidification process, or anti-acid program, which is described in this book. Doctors of holistic medicine have documented their success with deacidification treatment, and scientific studies have followed. (See the References section for further information.) Through this research, it's been realized that many a health complaint is the result of chronic acidosis and that this condition and its consequences can be prevented and reversed.

Acidosis as a cause of disease is not a new concept. It has been recognized as a contributing factor in many isolated conditions, including gout, heartburn, gastritis, and sore muscles.

However, acidosis's influence on the body as a whole and its role in multiple health complaints are becoming important considerations.

Despite numerous medical scientific publications, it is difficult to obtain understandable or useful information on acidosis. That's where this book comes in. In *The Acid Danger*, you'll find the basic ideas and facts about acidosis. You'll learn about the causes of this condition and steps you can take to cure or prevent the problem. The simple fact that you, as a reader, wish to acquaint yourself with acidosis elevates you to the level of those who wish to avoid misdiagnosis of disease and the resulting unsuccessful treatment. Reading this book identifies you as an open-minded and progressive person. And this is a promising precondition for a successful encounter in the fight against acidosis. It is now up to you to take control of your health. This book can provide you with the tools, but you must use them.

CHAPTER 1

Understanding Acidosis

The negative effects of acidosis are far reaching, both internally and externally. To gain a full understanding of acidosis, it is important to consider that it can affect every level of the human body, including mental outlook, overall metabolism, organs, tissues, cells, molecules, atoms, and chromosomes. It even affects the environment. Consider, for example, the effect of acid rain—acid precipitation caused by pollutants in the atmosphere. Acid rain contributes damage to forests, soil, and lakes and streams, thereby endangering the animals and plants that depend on them—including humans. If costly environmental measures aren't taken by various governments to reduce acid precipitation and to counter its effects, it is likely that we will be faced with dangerously few healthy forests and a depletion of food sources. This is obviously a serious problem, but our purpose is to focus on metabolic acidosis—the type that occurs when the body is out of balance. This chapter is designed to give you a basic understanding of the acid/alkaline balance in the body and how a shift in this balance can lead to acidosis.

THE ACID/ALKALINE BALANCE— FROM BIRTH TO DEATH

A proper acid/alkaline balance (also called pH balance) is essential to the creation of life. The vaginal canal is acidic, while seminal fluid is alkaline (or base). The environment of the vagina must be neutralized by the alkalinity of the seminal

THE PROBLEM OF OVERSIMPLIFYING THE CAUSE OF DISEASE

People tend to oversimplify matters when attempting to determine the cause of a disease or illness. Of course it's easier to attribute an illness to something that's obvious. For example, gout is a metabolic disease characterized by inflamed joints, deposits of urates (uric acid salts) around the joints, and an excessive amount of uric acid in the blood. This condition is caused by an excess of uric acid in the body, a form of acidosis. The gout medication Allopurinol is usually prescribed to slow the production of uric acid, but the cause of the high uric acid levels is neither researched nor alleviated with this treatment.

In an effort to truly achieve good health, the cause must be investigated more deeply. What caused the excess uric acid to build up in the first place, and how can it be counteracted? Some possible causes include overconsumption of purine-containing foods, such as beef, pork, and organ meets; overconsumption of alcohol; the presence of a tumor; a high intake of fatty foods; defects in certain enzymes; malfunctioning or weak kidneys; insufficient intake of water; insufficient intake of nutrients; or a combination of these things.

Unfortunately, standard medical treatment for gout often ignores these factors and actually encourages acidosis: The ailing gout patient may receive cortisone injections as well as injections of antirheumatic substances (which are mostly acids or acid salts) to alleviate the pain and inflammation. A patient may endure this treatment until the acid-equalizing mechanisms in the body are exhausted to the point of organ malfunction. It doesn't have to be this way. Lifestyle changes that involve deacidification, correct nutrition, and the elimination of unhealthy substances are key factors in regaining health in this and many other acid-related disorders.

fluid for the sperm to live long enough to reach their destination. If this neutralization is successful, the first battle against acidosis has been won. Shortly before a person dies, metabolism collapses and the acid/alkaline balance shifts toward the acidic. As soon as acid has the upper hand, the final battle is lost. In the interim, the body is constantly fighting against acids and warding off their attacks.

Health, as well as illness, depends to an extent on the chemical-biological-physical reaction mechanisms in which the acid/alkaline balance plays a central part. The human body has a complex system of "acid/alkaline regulation" so that acids and alkalis can work to its benefit. Several buffer systems control against the danger of slipping into either excess acidity or alkalinity and are discussed later in this chapter. This balance is an inherent part of all functional processes of the body and shows measurable changes in case of disease processes.

> ## METABOLISM
>
> *The range of chemical and physiological processes necessary for the maintenance of life through which the body breaks down nutrients, oxygen, and enzymes to produce energy for bodily functions; maintains and builds cells; and eliminates waste compounds. Acids have an essential role in metabolism.*

THE CONCEPT OF pH

All life processes take place in water. The water molecule has the chemical formula H_2O, which means that it is composed of two hydrogen atoms and one oxygen atom. The degree of acidity is an important chemical property of watery systems. Chemists describe the degree of acidity of a watery system as the concentration of water-bound hydrogen ions (H_3O^+ ions or H^+ ions for short). In pure water, the concentration of the positively charged acidic H^+ ions equals the concentration of the negatively charged basic OH⁻ ions. When the concentration of acidic ions equals that of basic ions, the solution is considered *neutral*. In fact, the concentrations of H^+ and OH^- ions in pure water are very low: Expressed in decimal figures, they each correspond to a number of 0.0000001 mass units per liter. In science, numbers with many zeros before or after the comma are more conveniently expressed as powers of ten (in our case, $1(10^{-7})$). In practice, concentrations of hydrogen ions in watery systems are nearly always expressed as the *negative* of the power to which ten must be raised to express the number (the p value). Since –7 is the power to which ten must be raised to express our concentration of H^+ ions, the p value would be –(–7) or simply 7. As it is a measure of the concentration of hydrogen ions, the corresponding p value is termed pH. See Table 1.1 for the average pH value of important body fluids.

Whether a liquid is acidic or alkaline depends on the direction in which the balance has shifted. If there are more acids than alkalis, the liquid lies within the acidic range. If the alkalis outweigh the acids, the environment is alkaline. Normally all systems work optimally within a specific range of pH value. An excess in either direction—acidic or alkaline—can harm these body systems. The illness is usually caused by a quiet or unobtrusive shift to the

pH VALUE

pH (which stands for potential of Hydrogen) is a measure of the acidity or alkalinity of a solution, based on the number of hydrogen ions in the liquid. The pH scale ranges from 0 (highest acidity) to 14 (highest alkalinity), with water having a neutral pH of 7. Since the pH is a logarithmic scale, every increase of 1.0 in measurement represents a tenfold increase in alkalinity, and a pH of 4 would be 100 times more acidic than a pH of 6. In essence, pH determines both acidity and alkalinity based on the presence or absence of hydrogen ions. The more hydrogen ions present, the more acidic the solution.

acidic range. Only in exceptional cases is a shift to the alkaline range reported. (Excessive alkalinity rarely occurs in the human body. This condition is known as alkalosis and has an array of symptoms that go beyond the scope of this book.)

TABLE 1.1. THE AVERAGE PH VALUE OF IMPORTANT BODY FLUIDS

Body Fluid	pH value	Body Fluid	pH value
Bile	7.5–8.8	Saliva	7.2–7.5
Blood	7.37–7.43	Seminal fluid	7.8–8.2
Gastric juices	2.5	Urine	6.2
Pancreatic juice	7.5–8.8	Vaginal secretion	4.0–4.7

It is easy to recognize from the different pH values how important the regulation of the acid/alkaline balance is. Not all acids are dangerous, but they must perform their activities in the right place at the right time. When systems become disturbed, the balance usually shifts in favor of the acids. This causes countless malfunctions of biological systems. Fortunately, a proper metabolism has many ways to regulate the acid/alkaline balance.

BIOLOGICAL REGULATORY SYSTEMS/ BUFFER SYSTEMS

The body has several options for maintaining the acid/alkaline balance. For example, the lungs can breathe out increased amounts of carbon dioxide (CO_2), when an excess is present. CO_2 dissolves in water to form carbonic acid. This breathing out of CO_2 is a short-term method to eliminate fugitive acids. Intensive-care units are on constant watch for the release of CO_2 by patients. As soon as the system slips and the levels of acids increase, a person's situation becomes critical and death can follow.

The kidneys eliminate acids via the urine. Because the kid-

THE MOST IMPORTANT ACIDS FOR THE HUMAN BODY

Many of the acids listed below are an essential part of metabolism in the human body. You may be more familiar with the names of some of these acids, such as amino acids and fatty acids, than you are with others. These body acids are responsible for the function of different enzymes (proteins that initiate biochemical reactions). If these acids are too strong or are working in the wrong system, they can cause serious harm to the body. Gastric acid, for example, is necessary for normal stomach functioning. If, however, too much gastric acid is produced, it will affect the stomach lining and lead to gastritis or even to stomach ulcers. Here's another example: Normal muscle functioning produces low quantities of lactic acid. If, however, the muscle is overexerted, excessive lactic acid will be produced, thus damaging the muscle cells. This results in aching muscles, a pain we all know.

Not all of the following acids are produced in the body. Some are found in drugs or food.

- Acetylsalicylic acid
- Acidic acid
- Amino acid
- Arachidonic acid
- Carbonic acid
- Fatty acids
- Hydrochloric acid

- Lactic acid
- Nitric acid
- Perchloric acid
- Phosphoric acid
- Prussic acid
- Sulphuric acid
- Uric acid

neys need water to perform this important function, drinking a sufficient amount helps this process along. (See Chapter 4 for some guidelines on water intake.)

The blood and blood plasma also are equipped with buffer systems. Thanks to nature, the blood buffer systems are the best-functioning defense mechanisms against acid attacks. The body tries to maintain a blood pH value at a constant level of between 7.37 and 7.43. A pH value of 7.4 means the blood is in an alkaline pH range. Properly functioning buffer systems combine appropriate alkalis with acids to maintain the proper balance. The most important buffer systems in our blood include the hemoglobin buffer, the phosphate buffer, the bicarbonate buffer, and the protein buffer.

The natural biological buffering (neutralization) mechanisms are limited by their capacity to take up acids and to neutralize acid excess. These mechanisms suffer enormously as a result of the environmental conditions and lifestyle of the twenty-first century, such as nutrition that is rich in animal protein and fat, stress, alcohol consumption, and age-related decline in kidney function. Although the body has equipped its systems perfectly, it is in the interest of your health to assist these systems by treating your body appropriately and not placing additional strain on them.

When these buffer systems are highly stressed but still have the ability to maintain a borderline blood-acid level, "silent" or "sneaking" acidosis (latent acidosis) has gained a foothold. As soon as the buffer reserves are depleted, the entire system is in danger of toppling over, which could set off numerous illnesses. The body is forced to deposit the acids somewhere, and these deposits can disturb individual body systems for years.

MEASURING ACIDOSIS

An entire branch of modern medical science is dedicated to the art of measuring and assessing, but these measurements aren't always reliable. Some assessments do not reflect the true metabolic situation within the entire body, since measuring one of the many bodily fluids merely represents a momentary picture of a complex system. The measured values of blood, urine, saliva, gastric juices, and so on do not necessarily reflect the complete acid/alkaline balance; other considerations have to be taken into account. For example, information about the condition of tissue in clinical examinations is more valuable to the experienced diagnostician than the long-term recording of the morning pH values of urine. It is, for instance, possible to determine acid levels by touching the tissue above the sacrum (the triangular bone that forms the posterior section of the pelvis). In case of excessive acids in the body, lumps in the connective tissue will often hurt when subjected to pressure. Moreover, it's possible to evaluate acid levels by examining the color and condition of skin and tongue. The information gathered from a case history might also suggest the presence of chronic acidosis, either as a cause or side effect of disease.

Although the measuring processes discussed below fall short in their ability to accurately prove the existence or nonexistence of acidosis, they are widely used to test for its existence. You should familiarize yourself with these tests, but know that the best indicator for the existence of acidosis is a general lack of well-being and a susceptibility to various illnesses. Acidosis is rarely detected in people of good health who are full of the joys of life.

Blood Processes

Blood samples are obviously required for blood processes, which generally require a fully equipped laboratory. Blood processes include blood-gas analysis, blood lactic acid assessment, blood buffer capacity assessment, blood uric acid assessment, and bodily fluid acid content assessment. Each of these processes is discussed in the following sections.

Blood-Gas Analysis

This process mainly measures the condition of arterial blood and is usually used in intensive medical science, where it is of great significance. However, a blood-gas analysis does not accurately reflect the total pH balance of the body. It only provides information about CO_2 acids, which indicate the condition of the lungs.

Blood Lactic Acid Assessment

The application of measured lactates lies mainly in the field of performance diagnosis and sports medicine, and some modern training methods are based entirely on this assessment method. The lactic acid test is useful for testing fitness, but does not necessarily provide adequate information for assessing total pH balance. This is because it takes into account only the presence of lactic acid and the capability of the muscles to neutralize it.

Blood Buffer Capacity Assessment

In this process, small quantities of acid are added in increments to full blood and blood plasma (blood without cells). The longer it takes for the pH value to decrease in value (become more acidic) in this process, the better the capacity of the blood to buffer excess acid.

Blood Uric Acid Level Assessment

This process provides a great deal of information about metabolism, since high levels of uric acid usually indicate a body-wide acid overload. However, a normal level of uric acid does not mean that there is no acid strain present in the body. For example, gout attacks are possible in people with normal lab levels of uric acid.

Bodily Fluid Acid Content Assessment

The most significant fluid is synovial fluid (a lubricant for joints and tendons). The presence of uric acid crystals or inflammatory amino acids is measured in this process, mainly in the joints of the knees, hips, and shoulders. This checkup is usually performed to investigate the cause of arthritis rather than to determine the acid/alkaline balance.

Non-Blood Processes

Individual urine measurements are often used to provide simple and inexpensive proof of acidosis, but the diagnostic value is arguable. The pH value of urine is subject to strong influences such as diet, and also depends largely on how much water one drinks. Urine is supposed to be acidic. A low pH value of urine merely indicates that the kidneys are excreting an increased amount of acid, which is a desirable process. Also, measuring urine does not indicate the effectiveness of the alkaline substances taken for a load test (see below).

Load Test by Way of Standardized Alkaline Substances (such as Alkaline Powder)

In this test, alkaline powder is taken after morning urine has been measured. The urine is then measured over the next few hours and should reflect an increase in the pH value. However, this value is also of little importance since the pH measurement of urine is subject to many different influences, as mentioned above.

In summary, the answer is a vague "Yes, but . . ." regarding the question of whether acidosis can be measured. Although the pH value of every fluid in the body can be measured, the relevance of this information is questionable. Individual tests are inadequate for measuring acidosis because each single result—be it blood, urine, saliva, or perspiration—paints only a temporary picture. The pH value of urine, for instance, is subject to so many factors that it becomes virtually meaningless. The only thing that can be measured is how much acid was excreted in the last urination. It is, to phrase it simply, impossible and irresponsible to deduct from a single measurement of urine whether latent acidosis is present or not.

Urine is physiologically slightly acidic. In the case of urinary tract infections, the pH value shifts toward the alkaline range (bacteria create an alkaline environment). The volume of water that's consumed can influence the relative acid content of urine significantly.

The various blood tests indicate the acid/alkali status of the plasma and the total blood regulation, but no definite statement can be made about the whole body. Strain and titration tests allow for conclusions about the buffer systems. They're also important measurements of the entire body, but unfortunately they, too, represent only a temporary situation. Other disadvantages are the price of the tests and the complicated procedures; the determination of uric acid is still regarded as relatively simple in comparison.

There is no a simple procedure yet to determine the complete state of acidosis in the body, but some tests, such as the determination of special kidney enzymes, raise hope for simpler procedures in the future. Another possibility is to examine the trace elements in the blood. Measuring selenium, zinc, magnesium, and calcium content are primary determinants for conclusions concerning the acid/alkali balance. Testing heavy metal levels can also proves helpful. An increased heavy metal level allows for an assumption of chronic acidosis, since loading with heavy metals increases acidosis.

In short, conclusions based only on measurements of the pH value of urine have to be rejected. A diagnosis of acidosis can be determined precisely and in its entirety only through the combination of a clinical analysis, several laboratory tests, and detailed questioning. An evaluation scale is in development for this purpose.

TYPICAL SYMPTOMS OF ACIDOSIS

Acidosis can become a problem at any age. If latent (or silent) acidosis is not treated, it can result in a variety of symptoms. Weakened kidneys from any cause at any age increase the likelihood that acidosis will develop, because the kidneys are responsible for filtering out acidic wastes. In any event, kidney function tends to slow and metabolic function becomes restricted as people age, resulting in an increase of acid attacks as well as insufficient elimination of acids. Someone who suffers from acidosis may be anywhere from severely underweight to seriously overweight and most likely suffers from a stiff spine as a result of the chronic inflammation of the intervertebral joints. The small joints of the hands and feet are probably also affected. Chronic pain is usually the norm. In many cases of chronic acidosis, a person may have had or will need at least three of the following operations:

- Gallbladder removal

- Tumor excision

- Full or partial resection of stomach

- Kidney stone removal

- Surgery on intervertebral disks

- Pancreas surgery (also called the Whipple operation)

- Joint replacement

- Colon surgery, mainly to remove tumors

The typical person suffering from chronic acidosis is frequently in a foul mood due to constant pain and perhaps a lack of mobility, which might lead to depression. In many cases the person has lost all hope of ever feeling better because he or she has tried various medical treatments and procedures without success.

A person with severe acidosis may have any or all of the conditions listed in Table 1.2. In fact, this table is a summary of almost every diagnosis in the entire medical field. You'll notice from this information that acidosis can be linked, either as a trigger or as a result, to almost every disease.

TABLE 1.2. POSSIBLE HEALTH PROBLEMS
ASSOCIATED WITH SEVERE ACIDOSIS

Gastrointestinal Tract

- Chronic or acute gastroenteritis
- Gallbladder problems
- Intestinal fungus
- Bloating
- Constipation
- Digestive problems
- Flatulence
- Foul-smelling feces

Muscles/Joints

- Gout
- Lower back pain
- Swollen legs
- Osteoporosis
- Muscle pain
- Osteoarthritis
- Damage to intervertebral discs
- Rheumatism in all its forms

Skin/Hair/Teeth

- Loss of hair
- Chronic rashes
- Brittle nails
- Various skin diseases
- Tooth decay
- Allergies
- Thinning gums
- Blemishes
- Dry skin
- Cellulite
- Skin fungus
- Acne

Metabolic System

- Overweight
- Kidney stones
- Ravenous hunger attacks
- Increased uric acid
- Diabetes
- Increased levels of liver enzymes, possibly indicating liver damage
- Weight gain
- Increased cholesterol level

Vascular System

- High blood pressure
- Poor circulation in legs
- Stroke
- Dizziness
- Calcification
- Migraines
- Coronary heart disease
- Heart attack

Entire Organism

- Suppressed immune system
- Lack of energy
- Chronic pains
- Nervousness
- Depression
- Inability to cope with stress
- General feeling of not being well
- Low libido
- Premature fatigue (so-called chronic fatigue syndrome)

RECOGNIZING ACIDOSIS IN YOURSELF

There's a difference between acute acidosis and quiet or latent acidosis. An acute acidosis is much less critical and more commonplace, and just leads to inflammation and pain such as gout, sore muscle, and gastritis. Chronic acidosis can cause a lot of different and much more severe diseases, and is therefore called a silent danger.

Acute acidosis affects everybody at regular intervals and occurs when you eat acid-forming foods, subject yourself to extremely intense physical strain, drink too much coffee or alcohol, and/or do not drink enough water. While acute acidosis can have symptoms, they are not present in all cases. Puffy eyes, gastroenteritis, joint problems, and many other symptoms can be signs that the metabolism is shifting temporarily into the acidic range. When these symptoms occur, an alkaline powder should be taken immediately to neutralize the excess acid in the body and avoid permanent damage to your health. (Keep in mind that over-the-counter antacids only neutralize gastric acid in the stomach and are used solely for treating gastritis, heartburn, or stomach ulcers. However, alkaline powder has an effect on the entire body. Not only does it neutralize gastric acid, but it also influences almost all other systems in the body.)

Dangerous latent acidosis can emerge if these symptoms are ignored. The acids or salts of the acid will place strain on your body's neutralization systems over the long term, which will, in turn, pose a serious threat to your health. The resulting illness usually depends on the individual and his or her lifestyle, but as a rule, the acids attack the weak points in the system.

Everyone suffers from acidosis at some stage in his or her life, but you can prevent the development of latent acidosis by applying correct measures. If you don't feel well and think it could be acidosis, start a deacidification treatment immediately. That way, the dangerous illnesses arising from acidosis can be treated or prevented. Those who suffer from acidosis for many years will require lengthy treatment to become deacidified. It is not unusual for a person to experience an unbelievable burst of energy as a result of deacidification.

ACIDOSIS IN BREASTFED INFANTS

A mother's nutrition considerably influences the well-being of her breastfed infant. A breastfed baby who has digestive problems may be suffering from acidosis. The process of deacidification in the mother can help alleviate such problems, which is why nursing mothers are usually advised to refrain from acidic and acid-forming food. (These foods are listed in Chapter 2.)

CONCLUSION

Maintaining a proper acid/alkaline balance within the body is vital for good health. The human body is a complex mechanism of systems that rely on a healthy metabolism to break down nutrients for energy and to remove wastes, and each of these systems must be within the proper pH level for optimal function. While an excess of either acidity or alkalinity can cause damage, the body's imbalances tend to be excess acidity. A healthy metabolism can handle occasional excess acid (acute acidosis) through its buffering mechanisms, but the long-term acid conditions of latent acidosis wears down these safeguards. Many people have no overt symptoms of latent acidosis, but since it is a condition that can be linked to every serious illness, it is essential to avoid. When you feel that you may have acute acidosis, treat it immediately with an alkaline powder. If you believe you may have latent acidosis, it is important to start deacidification treatment to avoid serious problems over time. Maintaining proper acid levels should be your primary step towards insuring your health. The next chapter will provide some preventive information regarding acid-causing foods and other factors to assist in avoiding acidosis.

CHAPTER 2

The Causes
of Acidosis

M any factors play a role in the development of acidosis. I've refrained from discussing the more complex patho-logical and pathophysiological factors to avoid lengthy sci-entific explanation and speculation. This chapter discusses a few universally common causes that have been established and are a good starting point for understanding the origin of this condition.

THE MOST COMMON CAUSES OF ACIDOSIS

One or more of the following factors can cause a person's metabolism to shift toward the acidic range. Acidosis can take a permanent hold if no actions are taken to counteract these changes and avoid further triggers.

Causes of acidosis include the following:

• Inadequate nutrition

• Use of addictive substances

• Inadequate intake of water

• Stress

• Side effects of certain medications

• Too little or too much physical activity

Although these causes apply in most cases of acidosis, they need not lead to illness. You can adapt your lifestyle in an attempt to neutralize the flood of acids attacking your body, but not doing anything to counteract the negative effects of acid buildup allows acidosis to become a chronic condition that will eventually lead to illness. The following discussions offer a closer look at each of these causes.

Inadequate Nutrition

Various factors influence the impact of nutrition on the acid/alkaline balance, so there are no universal rules regarding nutrition in the fight against acidosis. However, this doesn't eliminate the need to take a close look at nutrition and how it affects the body. Begin by asking yourself the important questions listed below. Just keep a mental note of your answers for now; in Chapter 3 we will revisit these questions and see how these answers can affect your metabolism of acids.

What do you eat?

How much do you eat?

When do you eat?

How often do you eat?

How well do you chew your food?

How well does your body digest your food?

How well does your body tolerate food?

How is your food produced?

Food Categories

In discussions of acidosis, food is generally broken down into four categories: acid-forming foods, acidic foods, alkaline foods, and alkali-forming foods. Each of these categories is discussed briefly below.

ACID-FORMING FOODS

These foods are not acidic themselves, but form acids in the body during the metabolic process and digestion.

The foods listed below produce acids or acidic substances

as a metabolic byproduct during their absorption and utilization by the body. This is a natural process necessary for digestion. However, you shouldn't eat too much of these foods or eat them too often. If too much meat or any other acid-forming foods are eaten, it is a good idea to counteract their effects by taking an alkaline powder (see Chapter 5) and also by abstaining from acid-forming foods for a few days. Below are some common acid-forming foods. Additionally, these foods contain *arachidonic acid,* which is responsible for rheumatic diseases (inflammation or pain in muscles, joints, or tissue):

- Animal fats
- Animal-based spreads
- Bacon
- Cheese
- Luncheon meats
- Beef

- Pork
- Organ meats
- Poultry
- Sausages
- Smoked meats

The following foods can also cause acidosis indirectly by forming acid in the body. These foods, however, do not contain arachidonic acid.

- Alcoholic beverages (mostly champagne)
- Fried fish
- Potato chips
- Chocolate
- Coffee
- Eggs
- Legumes

- Mayonnaise
- Mustard
- Peanuts
- Sugar
- Sweets
- Tea
- Tomato sauce

ACIDIC FOODS

These foods are acidic, but can have either an acid-forming or an alkaline-forming effect in the body.

The foods in this group are in themselves acidic. You can often feel the effect of these "acids" in your stomach after you've eaten foods from this category. Whether they have an acidic effect or an alkaline effect in further metabolic processes depends on various factors, including how they are combined with other foods (not necessarily other acidic foods) and when they are eaten. Frequently, the act of combining these foods is the cause of the burning sensations in the stomach. But *when* you eat these foods also determines the further development of acids. The following is a list of some common acidic foods:

- All sour-tasting foods and beverages

- Berries

- Citrus fruit

- Fresh cheese

- Fruit juices

- Pulses, such as lentils or peas

- Sour milk or cream

- Stone fruits (fruits with hard pits at their center, such as peaches, plums, and apricots)

- Unripe fruit

- Vinegar

ALKALINE FOODS AND ALKALI-FORMING FOODS

Both alkaline and alkali-forming food groups are discussed simultaneously, as there is no great difference between them. *The strength of the alkali in alkaline foods does not reflect their alkali-forming qualities in the body. Alkali-forming foods are not alkaline them-*

selves, but they possess good alkali-forming and deacidifying qualities.

A deacidification process cannot be performed merely through consuming more alkaline foods and beverages; it's simply too difficult to eat enough of these foods to make a difference. (If you don't counteract acids with an alkaline powder over the years as discussed in Chapters 4 and 5, acids and acid salts will undoubtedly accumulate in your body.) The following is a list of common alkaline and alkali-forming foods:

- Potatoes and potato juice

- Roots (such as carrots, turnips, and radishes)

- Alkaline milk products—regular milk is alkaline, sour milk, sour cream, and most cheeses are acid forming

- Most fresh vegetables

- Leafy salad greens

- Some fully ripened fruits, such as grapes and apples

- Spinach

- Bananas

- Celeriac

- Melons

Addictive Substances

The following section discusses the most common addictive substances used in our society today—coffee, nicotine, and alcohol. As you already know, these substances have many negative effects on the body, only one of which is acidosis. Overuse of these substances can lead directly to severe acidosis. While anyone who smokes should give up nicotine completely, those who consume alcohol and coffee in moderation can neutralize their acid-forming properties by taking alkaline powder (see Chapter 4 and 5) and by drinking plenty of water (see Chapter 4).

Coffee

As a consequence of the roasting process, coffee beans create excess acid in the body, which, in turn, often lead to excessive gastric acid and subsequently to gastroenteritis and ulcers. Drinking too much coffee can also result in heartburn. Moreover, caffeine increases the blood circulation of kidney marrow. Increased blood circulation of kidney marrow leads to increased diuresis (water excretion), creating yet another chance for acidosis to take hold.

If you don't want to give up coffee, drink a lot of plain water along with it to replenish the water you will lose. Switching to decaffeinated coffee can help you avoid the diuretic effect of caffeine.

Nicotine

The aggression of the hydrocarbons in cigarettes is very disturbing to the health of the body, and the acidic effect of cigarettes is underestimated. Nicotine stimulates the formation of gastrine, a hormone that encourages the secretion of gastric acid. This is why smokers are more prone to developing ulcers than nonsmokers. Nicotine has an effect on the kidneys similar to caffeine in that it withdraws liquid from the body. Nicotine also causes the production of a flood of stress hormones, such as adrenaline and noradrenaline. Long-term high stress levels can cause irreversible malfunctions throughout the body.

Alcohol

Alcoholic beverages are counted among the strongest acid-forming substances. This is due to the metabolic processing of alcohol in the liver rather than to the increased production of gastric acid, which was frequently the assumption in the past. It's easy to understand why you have a hangover after a night on the town; hangover symptoms are a result of acute acidosis. Dehydration occurs along with the acidosis, creating that characteristic thirst during a hangover.

Inadequate Water Intake

Experience has shown that many people who suffer from acidosis simply do not drink enough water. Water plays an important role in the neutralizing process and acid excretion and is vital in flushing out common salt from the body. The quality of drinking water is an influencing factor in its ability to assist the body in these processes, and also determines the nature of thirst (that is, the natural urge to drink water). Pure thirst, or a natural desire for plain water, has virtually disappeared over the last few decades due to the intense taste of most of today's beverages, as well as to our lifestyle. (See Chapter 4 for guidelines on water intake and more information about water quality and purity.)

Stress

Without fail, physical stress and mental stress lead to an enormous acidosis problem. These hormonally and biologically controlled metabolic processes produce acid as a natural reaction to stress, and strain the body when it becomes a chronic condition. A few of the most common stress hormones are cortisol, adrenaline, and noradrenaline. Most of the systems in the body will accelerate metabolic processes when they are subjected to high levels of stress hormones. This, in turn, leads to increased acid accumulation in the organs. Being under constant stress leads to the "stress habits" listed below. These stress habits further cause the body to become overly acidic.

Stress Habits

- Cigarette smoking
- Eating too quickly
- Performing sports activities too intensely or incorrectly
- Not taking in the proper nutrients
- Habitually worrying, feeling anxious, or experiencing inner turmoil

- Not taking in sufficient water

- Sleeping poorly

- Failing to take adequate leisure time

- Overconsuming alcohol

- Overconsuming coffee

Side Effects of Medication

Nonsteroidal antirheumatics (NSAR), such as mefenamic acid and diclofenac acid, are often prescribed for people with rheumatism, which as you've learned is an acid-related illness characterized by pain in muscles, joints, or fibrous tissue. While such medications certainly have a role in the short-term relief of pain, the question arises whether an acid-related illness (rheumatism) can be cured with an acid in the long term. Some of the most frequent side effects of NSARs are gastroenteritis, ulcers, and even gastric hemorrhages. Sometimes an additional medication is given to slow down the production of gastric acid to avoid gastric upset. This medication, in turn, encourages body-wide acidosis.

The healthcare industry would save billions of dollars every year if deacidification were used as an initial treatment in the case of rheumatic disorders such as lower back pain and joint pain, and if immediate and long-term therapy with acidic medication were avoided. This also applies to aspirin, one of the most successful and most widely used medications. The pharmacological name of aspirin is acetylsalicylic acid. This acid blocks prostaglandin synthesis and interferes with the acid in the acid/alkaline balance.

> **PROSTAGLANDINS**
>
> *A class of hormonelike fatty acids in mammalian tissues and cells that are involved in many body processes, including inflammation, smooth muscle function, pain, blood pressure, kidney function, gastroduodenal protection, and childbirth labor.*

Aspirin is not only used as an antirheumatic or pain relief medication, but is also taken for cases of flu or bronchitis. The symptoms of a cold are very similar to the symptoms of acute acidosis. Simply drinking enough water will relieve flu symptoms considerably. Alkaline powder brings additional relief (see Chapter 5).

If you are in doubt about whether or not a medication you take causes excess acid to build up in your body, ask a qualified health professional.

Lack of Physical Activity

Lack of excise greatly influences the acid/alkaline balance. A lack of physical activity has a serious effect on the acid/alkaline balance. This is particularly recognized in Europe, where alkaline powder has been used very successfully to correct acidosis due to inactivity. Light movement improves metabolism because it burns fatty acids as well as other acids. It also stimulates liver enzymes to burn fatty acids. This deacidification mechanism—the burning process in muscle tissue—is often neglected by overweight people who tend to get inadequate exercise. Also, a lack of physical activity creates a slight increase in weight, and excess weight, in turn, encourages acidosis. And the cycle starts anew.

Too Much Physical Activity

Intense physical stress results in an excess of lactic acid and other acids in the muscles. Athletes who overtrain—that is, they don't take "rest days," which would give lactic acid levels a chance to return to normal—are in short-term jeopardy of developing hernias and other muscle injuries, and are in for more serious problems in the long run. From the viewpoint of the sports physician, the formation of lactates (salts of lactic acid) should be prevented. Look for alkaline powders specifically developed for the needs of an athlete at pharmacies. These increase the lactate tolerance of muscle cells and enhance the performance of the muscle. Excessive physical activity at the workplace can also be a problem. For example, after thirty years on the job, a construction worker will most likely be suffering from joint damage as a result of chronic acidosis.

CONCLUSION

The causes of acidosis mentioned in this chapter certainly do not form an exhaustive list. Acidosis can occur in many different ways and is a permanently lurking danger in everyday life—while eating, drinking, fasting, working, playing sports, and in the aging process. Fortunately, if you are aware of the causes, you'll be better able to avoid the dangers of acidosis. The consequences of ignoring acidosis can be understood more clearly through the information provided in the next chapter.

CHAPTER 3

The Consequences of Acidosis

Most biological systems are weakened, affected, or damaged by excess acid. The effects of general acidosis vary from person to person; there may be only one symptom or several simultaneous symptoms. A person's habits and characteristics determine the problem areas where the acids will attack. For example, a person who smokes many cigarettes a day is likely to develop stomach problems since nicotine increases the production of gastric acid—not to mention the many other risks associated with smoking. This chapter discusses the far-reaching consequence of acidosis, from its effects on individual systems to its effects on the entire organism—the human body.

EFFECTS ON THE GASTROINTESTINAL TRACT

The sixteenth-century physician Paracelsus said that the cause of all evil lies in the intestines, and it is a proven fact that many a health problem originates in the intestines and digestive tract. Innumerable toxins are produced when digestion is poor, and they flood the body. One of these toxins is excess acid.

The most obvious illnesses caused by acid affect the esophagus and the stomach. Even doctors who are unwilling to expand their knowledge recognize acidosis as a cause of disease in this instance.

Heartburn develops through the influence of acid in the lower part of the esophagus. The esophageal tissue is digested by the gastric juice, and this results in extensive ulcers. The same happens to the gastric lining if it is not protected against too much acid. Antirheumatic medications hinder the body's natural protection of the gastric lining and enable the gastric juices to attack the cells of the stomach's inner wall. These attacks can result in gastroenteritis (stomach inflammation), esophagitis (inflammation of the esophagus), *ulcus ventriculi* (stomach ulcer), and *ulcus duodeni* (duodenal ulcer).

The pancreas plays a significant role in digestion. If it doesn't produce sufficient alkalis to neutralize hydrochloric acid in the stomach, digestive problems such as duodenal ulcer or constipation will occur. The pancreas becomes overstressed by incorrect nutrition, and either gives up after years of futile effort or becomes limited in its performance. When the pancreas does not function properly, the results are constipation, a bloated feeling, flatulence, and a swollen abdomen.

Likewise, diseases resulting from intestinal fungi are significant in cases of acidosis. Although intestinal fungi such as yeast and other fungal toxins are normally present in our intestinal tract in small amounts, they are usually kept in check by the intestine's beneficial microflora (bacteria). An overproliferation of fungi (for example, *Candida albicans* and aflatoxin) can cause a number of illnesses. They're at home in an acid intestinal environment, and for this reason, the fungi ensure that the intestines provide an excess of acid by interfering with digestion, which leads to food decomposition in the intestines, resulting in foul gases. Intestinal fungi cannot be treated successfully without a deacidification process. In this case, no research studies are available because intestinal fungi are not treated in a medical clinic, but with natural remedies.

Although the liver is rarely discussed in cases of acidosis, its importance must not be underestimated. As the central metabolism and detoxification organ, the liver is far more important for the acid/alkaline balance than generally assumed. These correlations are currently being studied in medical clinics and their importance is being recognized. In the case of a hepatic coma (liver failure), there's a significant shift in the pH balance toward the acid range. The liver is already extremely stressed as a result of environmental and food toxins. Reducing the intake of acid-forming substances and taking alkaline powder can help to regenerate the liver.

If excessive alcohol consumption has damaged the liver, alcohol intake should be reduced or eliminated. In this case the liver will need assistance in its detoxification process, since the removal of undesirable metabolic toxins is most effective in an alkaline environment. Alkaline powder is widely used as a remedy for a hangover for this reason; it fights the acidosis caused by too much alcohol and helps the liver to regenerate.

EFFECTS ON MUSCLES, JOINTS, AND SPINE

Illnesses of the spine, joints, and muscles are frequently accompanied by relatively severe acidosis. The diseases will recur as long as this condition is not remedied. The most painful example of such illnesses is a gout attack. Uric acid settles in a joint in the form of uric acid crystals and causes severe inflammation. The uric acid burns as a fierce fire in the inflammation. In the case of joint and tissue rheumatism, this fire does not burn as fiercely, although it can continue for years.

If acidosis is not cured, most therapies are not permanently effective for many spinal diseases from the neck to the buttocks. This becomes obvious in massage therapy, which does not yield the desired results without deacidification. The acid deposits and salts can be felt in the muscles of the upper back and neck, and become palpable in the form of knobs and nodules above the sacrum. The lower back and the joints are areas where many people feel the effect of incorrect food consumption. The combination of excess weight from poor diet and resulting excess acid cause joint problems, which become one body-stressing entity initiating further acidity and damage.

The body can be damaged so badly from various types of excess acid development that the individual can experience years of suffering and even destruction of the joints. Quite frequently large deposits are stored in the body, and their removal and excretion takes a long time because the deacidification process must take place over a long period.

Arachidonic acid plays a central part in rheumatism. A study carried out at the University of Graz, Austria, showed that the level of arachidonic acid is clearly increased in patients who suffer from chronic rheumatism. Also, the amount of the arachidonic acid correlates with the intensity of pain. Arachidonic acid occurs in certain foods in a concentrated form and can cause inflammation. See the list on page 21 in Chapter 2 to review the foods that contain arachidonic acid.

Osteoporosis—decreased bone mass that primarily affects older women and people with weak kidneys—is a typical illness caused by acidosis. Chronic overloading with acids severely affects alkaline-reacting mineral substances such as calcium in the body and reduces their presence considerably. The result is a demineralization process particularly affecting the bone tissue. A negative calcium balance (the withdrawal of calcium from the bone) is the result of acidosis. When a bone or an egg is placed in vinegar—a common experiment in elementary school—after some time, the calcium will be eliminated by the acid in the vinegar. The result is a supple bone or rubbery eggshell. As osteoporosis develops, bone density decreases. Therefore, alkaline supplements (see Chapters 4 and 5) are advisable for all women.

EFFECTS ON SKIN, HAIR, AND TEETH

The factors that lead to the demineralization of the hair, nails, and teeth are similar to the factors that lead to osteoporosis. Increased zinc consumption together with an alkaline supplement can help in many cases of hair loss and brittle nails. (Zinc has no direct influence on acid/alkaline balance, but it does improve hair growth). Brittle and premature gray hair is an additional sign of excess acid.

People who have psoriasis (a chronic skin condition characterized by red patches with white scales) are usually well aware of the relationship between harmful acid-forming food and their skin condition. Alcohol increases the formation of scales considerably. Excessive acids accumulate in and around skin cells and cause inflammation, which, in turn, causes psoriasis through its keratinizing (process where fibrous keratin protein is deposited in cells, causing them to become horny) scale formation.

The cause is a bit more differentiated in an inflammatory skin condition called neurodermatitis. Allergic components and certain food incompatibilities are the release mechanisms of the inflammation. The affected person has often gone through a range of unusual diets and treatments with little effect, but many patients have confirmed the effectiveness of deacidification treatment. Parents report considerable improvement of the skin condition of children after a deacidification process combined with the proper nutritional principles. For example, after having tried all the different therapies to cure neurodermatitis in her child, a mother reported that her child had finally been cured with deacidification and continued observation of the basic rules for maintaining a proper acid/ alkaline relationship.

Scientific experience in the physiological and biochemical fields indicates that some acids produced by people with neurodermatitis cannot be excreted through the kidneys. These acids try to pass through the skin. They penetrate the skin cells but cannot exit completely and thus cause the undesirable inflammation. It's therefore especially important for people with neurodermatitis to drink enough water. Water helps to excrete these acids through the kidneys and helps the skin sweat, which also helps eliminate acids. (See Chapter 4 for a discussion on water intake.)

Even blemished skin, dry skin, and greasy skin can lead to the assumption that a person has metabolic problems. In the past, acne in youths and adults has been attributed to too much chocolate, sweets, and other dietary mistakes. We know today that most of these foods are acid-forming, so the cause of acne is to be found again in acidosis. Another factor in the case of skin problems is the pollution of the intestines, which is often linked to a fungus infection. Cellulite (lumpy, dimpled fat usually found in the thighs, hips, and buttocks) is also a problem that can be linked to faulty metabolism of fatty acids.

The skin is the most visible organ of the body and is constantly in contact with the environment. That makes it sensitive to acid attacks. A healthy lifestyle is extremely important for this organ, which reflects the state of your health to the outside world. Who does not want a clear skin?

Dentists report good results from deacidification therapy for the treatment of various forms of paradentosis (thinning of the gums) as well as for mouth ulcers. The tongue offers the experienced diagnostician a good means for establishing the acid/alkaline level, due to changes in color and texture. It is necessary to have some experience of diagnosis to see how strong the acidosis is. A taste that forms in the mouth can say a lot about the condition of the metabolism: A dry mouth with a bad taste is an alarm signal for acidosis.

EFFECTS ON METABOLISM

This book discusses metabolic diseases only briefly because their causes and the correlations between them are highly complex. For example, the metabolic disease diabetes mellitus affects almost all of the body organs, including the kidneys, heart, liver, and eyes. Specific details are beyond the scope of this book, but some basic points are covered below.

Gout

In the condition of gout, there's an increase in uric acid in the body, which can originate in various ways and in large quantities. This excess uric acid leads mostly to the formation of uric acid crystals. These are deposited in the joints, particularly in the big toes, where they cause severe inflammation and extreme pain. The pain is so severe that the person affected cannot even bear a blanket on his or her toes. Gout may affect other joints as well.

Other severe illnesses such as osteoarthritis, weak kidneys, and kidney stones can also occur through uric acid excess over many years. These illnesses destroy the joints and cause kidney stones and kidney damage. Fortunately this does not occur often if proper medical care, including deacidification treatment, is available.

Diabetes

Non-insulin-dependent diabetes (type 2) reflects the fatigue of the pancreas. The pancreas does not produce enough insulin or is unable to use it properly, resulting in increased blood-sugar levels. This increased blood-sugar level is the forerunner of many additional health problems that appear after years of high sugar levels, including eye problems, weak kidneys, heart problems, arteriosclerosis, and high blood pressure. These problems are usually linked to acidosis—that is, if high-blood sugar levels remain untreated, an abnormal accumulation of ketone bodies (ketosis) will cause chronic acidosis. (The worst complication of diabetes is called *ketoacidosis coma*—fainting as a result of acute acidosis through ketone bodies.) The abnormal accumulation of ketone bodies can be controlled by optimizing sugar values and by supplying certain minerals that neutralize acid, such as calcium and magnesium. (The best mixture for an alkaline powder is discussed later in the book.)

An additional factor in type-2 diabetes is that acid levels increase with each passing year, as the body's ability to disintegrate acids diminishes and the excretion system no longer functions at full capacity.

Excess Weight

In contrast to earlier opinions, being overweight is no longer regarded as a lack of discipline but rather as a malfunction of metabolism, in which the acid/alkaline balance plays an important role. This is discussed further in the next section.

EFFECTS ON WEIGHT

Whenever we see or smell food, the brain informs all of our organs that there will soon be something to eat and that they have to prepare for it. The salivary glands, stomach, pancreas, and liver start preparing for digestion. The cells lining the stomach produce hydrochloric acid. This production is reported to the brain and causes a strong feeling of hunger or, in some cases, an uncontrollable ravenous hunger. The stomach also sends a message to the pancreas to start producing alkaline substances as a protection mechanism to neutralize the excess gastric acid, so that it is not damaged by its own gastric acid. This kicks off the digestive processes in the small intestine. This metabolic process also causes a strong feeling of hunger that can, in some cases, become uncontrollable.

A simple example can be demonstrated with a slab of chocolate: A survey among Swiss chocolate producers shows that 80 percent of all chocolate eaters are determined to eat only one piece and then stop. This one piece starts off the above-mentioned metabolic processes and the hunger becomes uncontrollable. After a few minutes, nothing is left of the chocolate slab (including all of the calories!). The same mechanism applies to puddings, chips, salted nuts, snacks, and many other sweets, as these types of food produce a relatively high quantity of gastric acid without satisfying hunger.

These mechanisms can be counteracted by deacidification and improvement of the body's buffer systems. When buffer systems in the body are provided with sufficient minerals, this excessive acid production of the stomach can be stopped at an early stage and gastric acid will only be produced for a short time. That is, the feeling of hunger can be dampened or suppressed completely through neutralization in the early stages of the process. The chain is disrupted and that leads to a further reduction in hunger, which leads to weight loss.

To lose weight, take alkaline powder fifteen to twenty minutes *before* meals, preferably with plenty of water. This helps the body achieve acid/alkaline balance and purifies the body's systems. The body immediately loses a few pounds in weight through the purification process alone, resulting in a loss of common salt (sodium) and associated retained water. Thereafter, the process slows down as the fatty deposits are addressed. The metabolism and disintegration of fat involves a chemical and biological reaction that produces fatty acids, which are biodegraded in the liver. Acidosis is a forerunner of excess weight because it significantly blocks this breakdown process.

Although fat takes longer to burn, the process of weight loss continues as the cause of the excess weight is eliminated. To reduce weight, it is absolutely necessary to observe the basic rules of deacidification therapy.

The fight against acidosis also helps the body's ability to efficiently metabolize fat, which happens to such an extent that the level of cholesterols as well as triglycerides decreases. This illustrates once again the value of a healthy lifestyle: the elimination or lessening of most risk factors.

EFFECTS ON VASCULAR AND CIRCULATORY SYSTEM

Diseases of the cardiac vessels are caused by long-term acidosis. There is a good reason why a heart attack can be caused by acid-forming behaviors such as smoking, not drinking enough water, stress, increased blood fats, too much coffee, high blood pressure, and alcohol abuse, as explained below.

Acidosis causes premature calcification of the blood vessels through damage inflicted on the inner vascular walls, and also is responsible for the same processes in the brain. A stroke is the pinnacle of acid attacks on your brain vessels. Most strokes can be prevented if the basic principles of deacidification therapy are followed. Deacidification can often reduce dizziness, a preliminary stage of this common illness. Dizziness is caused by a less serious, early form of circulatory problems in the brain.

Other forms of functional vascular disturbances such as reduced blood flow in the extremities, migraine, and weakness of the veins are also aggravated by acidosis.

EFFECTS ON THE ENTIRE ORGANISM

The biological and biochemical interrelations cannot be illustrated as clearly when it comes to the entire body, since they concern the entire organism rather than individual metabolic symptoms. Medicine should always treat the entire human being, but doctors often ignore this basic principle simply because they have too much detailed knowledge of specific systems. In certain diseases involving the entire system, we refer to the testimonials of people who underwent deacidification. In Europe alone, millions of people have tried deacidification therapy. An old quote says: "Whoever heals is right!"

The body's defense system becomes badly damaged when the metabolism had been in the acidic range for too long. Athletes can confirm this, as they often suffer from infectious diseases after too much physical exertion. Their immune systems have been weakened by lactic acid and become susceptible to germs that cause various illnesses. This, in turn, causes a considerable relapse in their training condition and leads to a decrease in performance. Conversely, athletes and nonathletes alike often report that they experience tremendous "energy bursts" after deacidification.

Chronic pain, as well as depression, combined with loss of the enjoyment of life can be treated with deacidification therapy.

Acidosis can be a cause, an effect, or even a symptom of almost every illness. It should not be underestimated under any circumstances. Illnesses may be relieved with standard medical therapy in the short term; however, they can only be cured if the cause is eliminated. Undergoing a deacidification process brings about an improvement in the prognosis, especially in combination with a conservative or naturopathic treatment.

CONCLUSION

Excess acid adversely affects all biological systems. The body systems harmed in a particular person will depend upon that individual's particular strengths and weaknesses, but in the long run, acidosis has potentially severe consequences and will cause illness. No particular system is immune from damage: It can harm the organs of the gastrointestinal tract, causing diseases in the esophagus, the stomach, the pancreas, the liver, and the intestines. It is responsible for many illnesses of the muscles, joints, and spine, including osteoporosis and rheumatism. It harms the skin, hair, and teeth, and causes metabolic issues that can result in gout, diabetes, and weight problems, a factor in many other diseases. Acidosis affects the vascular system and is associated with brain and blood vessel problems. Not least, it negatively affects the body as a whole, impacting everything from athletic performance to one's general outlook on life. All of the above can be improved with deacidification therapy, so it is critical that we address acidosis as a preventive measure and to cure existing cases. The next chapter provides the tools you need for this.

CHAPTER 4

Curing and
Preventing Acidosis

Common sense tells us that eliminating the cause of an illness is the most important step toward the cure. Many
therapy methods fail because they merely treat the symptoms
rather than the causes of the illness. The key to successfully
curing disease is quite frequently found in neutralizing excess
acids or, better still, in preventing their development.

The chances of success in any therapy are increased if the
body can be assisted in the deacidification process. Excess acid
not only damages your health, but also hampers the effectiveness of numerous medications and naturopathic treatments.
The battle against excess acid is important in achieving well-
being and maintaining health. This includes a change of lifestyle and habits, as well as supplementing your diet with
alkaline substances.

If acidosis has manifested itself, the time is now to start a
deacidification process that includes lifestyle changes and taking alkaline supplements as part of your daily regimen. Now
is also the best time to start your acidosis prevention program—even if you don't think you're in danger of acidosis.
Don't be fooled into thinking acidosis can be avoided or cured
with a quick fix. The acid danger is everywhere, and you will
need to protect yourself for the rest of your life. This chapter
can get you started.

THE DEACIDIFICATION PROCESS

We all know how difficult it is to start a new and healthy life

41

when our unhealthy habits have become second nature. Few people can change their lifestyles overnight; so don't be worried if you can accomplish only small changes at a time. Start by implementing some of the basic rules for maintaining a proper acid/alkaline balance:

1. Practice correct nutrition.

2. Drink plenty of pure water.

3. Avoid addictive substances.

4. Exercise regularly, but do not overexercise.

5. Reduce the stress in your life by setting priorities.

6. Increase your well-being by listening to your needs.

7. Take alkaline powder to counteract the effects of acid.

When you've practiced these rules for a while and they've begun to replace your old habits, you will notice that something has changed: You will instinctively know what is and what is not healthy for you. The tools you need to practice these tenets are detailed below.

Practice Correct Nutrition

Good digestion is essential in maintaining a good acid/alkaline balance; the digestive system is a primary means for removing excess acid from the body. Correct nutrition is required for a properly functioning digestive system. Take another look at the categories of foods in Chapter 2. This is important information, but remember that *what* we eat is less important than *when* and *how* we eat. Many factors determine the category of different foods, but these factors go beyond the nutritional makeup of a particular food. For example, an individual's metabolism plays a large part in how he or she will react to and be able to digest different foods. A strong young man can get away with eating things that would not be good for an eighty-year-old diabetic woman. It is up to you to consider how your body reacts to different foods. Be aware that all of the following factors affect your body's reaction to the food you eat:

1. The amount of food you eat

2. The state of your metabolism

3. The method of food preparation

4. The state of your digestive system

5. What time you eat

6. Your age

7. The ingredients in the food

8. Your physical makeup

9. Your chewing habits

10. The current physical strain on your body

There is no such thing as a single diet that is ideal for everyone, as you can see from the factors that affect your body's reaction to the foods you eat. No matter what their category, certain foods are beneficial to different people at different times.

THE TOP FIVE DIETARY MISTAKES

1. Eating too fast

2. Eating too many fatty foods

3. Eating too much

4. Eating too late

5. Eating too often

What to Eat

In general, reduce your intake of acid-forming foods (listed in Chapter 2). Limit meat and other fatty foods to once a week. Don't go overboard trying to eat only alkali-forming foods; they are only effective at countering acid when they are eaten in unrealistically huge quantities.

Follow your instincts and eat only those foods you know will not cause you any digestive discomfort. Any food allergies you may experience from a certain food should be noted and that food should be avoided as much as possible.

Avoid fast food and ready-prepared meals. Be sure to eat only natural, high-quality foods even if it takes extra time to prepare healthy meals.

When to Eat

When you eat is very important for your digestion and metabolism. Always start the day with a solid breakfast. Your body will have enough time to digest and utilize the food until the next meal. Eating before bed is poor practice—especially if it is something like ripened fruit, which will ferment in the digestive tract. You should allow yourself at least two to three hours to digest your food before retiring. Be sure to time your meals properly so this can happen. Also, be sure to eat easily digestible foods, such as carbohydrates, for your last meal of the day.

How Much to Eat

The average person eats too much, and the resulting excess weight poses a serious threat to health and well-being. The simplest road to health is eating less, and this is easily accomplished by not waiting until you feel full to stop eating. Instead, stop shortly before you feel full, when you know you've eaten a sufficient amount, since it takes time for your stomach to tell the brain that it's full. Your body will get used to this new way of eating in a very short time, and you will feel satisfied sooner.

The "how much to eat" question does not only refer to total food consumption, but also to the quantity eaten at each meal. As you know, intake of acid-forming foods should be reduced, but small amounts can easily be neutralized with alkaline powder. For example, a rack of ribs should certainly be avoided but a modest piece of roast pork can be eaten safely by neutralizing its acid-forming effects with alkaline powder.

How Often to Eat

Eat only when you feel hungry. Eating times are usually pre-scheduled—breakfast, lunch, and dinner, with occasional snacks between meals. Don't fall into this habit of making mealtimes so rigid that you are eating simply because everyone else is. Wait until you are hungry even if it means putting aside some food for yourself while others are eating. Also, if you choose to snack during the day, choose foods that aren't acid forming.

How to Eat

The manner in which you eat is crucial for the enjoyment of your food and your body's ability to digest it properly. Be sure to implement the following guidelines to prevent acidosis or to counter its negative effects on your body and well-being:

1. Do not rush through your meals. Take enough time to eat at a leisurely pace.

2. Eat with hunger and joy—that is, wait until you are hungry and appreciate your food.

3. Be sure your food is tasty, but not unhealthful.

4. Chew your food well before swallowing to aid digestion.

5. Stop eating *before* you feel full.

6. Give your body time to digest your food before retiring for the night or before exercising.

7. Attach great value to the quality of your food and avoid processed foods whenever possible.

8. Neutralize acid-forming foods with alkaline powder.

9. Eat a balanced diet that works with your individual metabolism.

10. Eat only small amounts of sugar and fatty foods, including meat.

Since so many factors are involved in practicing proper nutrition, each person is responsible for finding his or her own road to "correct" foods. The most important factor in combating acidosis is a new approach toward your eating habits. The significance of digestion in the acid/alkaline balance must be taken into account whenever you eat.

Drink Plenty of Pure Water

Water is life.
Water is precious.
Water is vital in the deacidification process.

Because we've become so used to drinking artificially sweetened beverages, we've almost lost our natural sensation of thirst. We must retrain ourselves to drink plenty of pure water because acidosis cannot be cured or prevented without doing so. Even the best alkaline powder cannot help to deacidify your body and prevent diseases if you don't drink enough water.

What is considered plenty? The minimum amount is 64 to 80 ounces of pure water a day. Of course, ideal water consumption depends on physical demands, body temperature, general activity, metabolism, age, and many other factors. In case of fever and infectious diseases, the demand for water increases threefold. Also, approximately one liter (approximately 35 ounces) of water needs to be replaced for every one hour of physical activity.

Most acids that occur in the body are excreted by the kidneys, and the kidneys need water to do this—preferably pure, high-quality mineral water that's low in sodium and carbonic acid. The worldwide success of the French mineral water Evian is probably based mainly on the fact that it is low in sodium.

It isn't always possible to drink a sufficient amount of water, simply because the water has to leave the body again. It's unpleasant to have to run off to the restroom constantly. However, at least once a day, try to drink enough water so that your urine is almost clear.

In most cases, the ingredients of traditional beverages such as alcohol and coffee produce more acid than can be excreted by the body. Therefore, if you drink alcohol, drink several glasses of water with each alcoholic drink, and when you drink a cup of coffee, drink two glasses of water. Half a liter (about 18 ounces) of water neutralizes the diuretic effect of a small cup of coffee and thus prevents acidosis.

Avoid Addictive Substances

Limit your consumption of alcohol to a sensible quantity. Consume wine or beer in small quantities if you wish, but always accompany these beverages with plenty of water. If you drink wine, choose red over white since red contains less acid. In small quantities, red wine is alkaline-forming, but in large quantities, it forms acid.

Due to the high concentration of alcohol, hard liquor such as whisky, brandy, gin, vodka, and rum should be avoided altogether. If even a small glass of whisky is drunk after an evening meal, for example, it must be neutralized the next day by avoiding all acid-producing foods and beverages, drinking plenty of water, and taking alkaline powder.

Nicotine and other tobacco products should also be avoided. Unfortunately, nicotine is particularly addictive and every ex-smoker knows how difficult it is to go without a cigarette. The acidic effect of nicotine is known and indisputable, and was partially discussed earlier. Smokers in particular have an enormous need for alkalis, and therefore must take alkaline substances on a regular basis. Smokers do not merely become ill as a result of acidosis, but also age faster.

Caffeine is another popular addictive substance. There is nothing to be said against coffee, provided it's consumed in small quantities. However, coffee consumption must be neutralized by the additional consumption of plain water (one cup of coffee needs to be neutralized by 16 ounces of water) and by the use of alkaline powder.

Get Regular Exercise, But Don't Overexercise

Physical activity can be deacidifying, but the activity must be performed correctly. The accumulation of lactic acid must be avoided through controlled training. Never exercise so intensely that you feel unable to perform the same task again afterward. Extreme physical strain damages the body. It is important to the deacidification process to select the correct level of physical exertion for the specific activity. You can do this by practicing the following:

1. Feel well in each phase of training.

2. Don't exert yourself too much.

3. Make sure you perspire.

4. Enjoy the activity.

Suffering from the effects of too much lactic acid (for example, sore muscles and a weakened immune system) is a clear indication that an athlete has been exerting himself too much. To remedy this, the athlete should exert himself less during training and also improve his buffer capacity with the use of alkaline powder. Nonathletes are simply advised to go for long walks or hikes. To reiterate, after exercising, a person should feel able to repeat the same exercise again without any major effort. If nonathletes desire to become involved in other exercise routines or sports, they should increase the frequency and intensity of exercise gradually and never subject their bodies to too much lactic acid.

Sweating in a sauna, steam bath, or bathtub is also recommended as some acids, such as sour manganese salts, leave the body mainly through the skin, and forced sweating enhances this process. (An unpleasant body odor occurs when the acid-releasing mechanism is disrupted, resulting in an excess of this acid retained in the body.) Don't forget to replace the water you lose in your sweat with plenty of fresh water. For example, for every fifteen minutes you are in a sauna, drink an additional 16 ounces of water.

Reduce the Stress in Your Life by Setting Priorities

Stress reduction leads to increased well-being. Consider the benefits of tranquility and serenity, and keep in mind the old proverb: "In our youth we chase after money with our health, and in our old age, we chase after health with our money." Set priorities in your life. Eliminate activities that you find unfulfilling or taxing. Learn to say no to others when you don't want to do something, and take that time to do something that brings you joy. Take steps to reduce work-related stress and lifestyle stressors. Take frequent breaks from your day-to-day routines—your body and your psyche will benefit. If you feel stressed out, slow down and relax.

Increase Your Well-Being By Listening to Your Needs

Without a doubt, the most important factor for a healthy and contented life is simply your well-being. Well-being is measured in different ways in different people. One person enjoys idleness; another does not. You may want to laze around and take it easy today, but tomorrow you may want to actively seek out adventure. It is important to listen to your needs and to give in to them. But be honest with yourself about what your needs really are. Daily well-being should become your constant aim— today, here, and now. Don't postpone this until retirement.

Maintain a Proper Acid/Alkaline Balance with Alkaline Supplements

Adding alkaline powder (also called base powder) to your regular supplement regimen will help you to neutralize excess acids in your body and will help to compensate for any malfunctions in your metabolism of acids. Alkaline powders have long been used in Europe to combat acidosis with great success.

It is best to take a standardized registered alkaline powder from a reputable manufacturer. In my experience, alkaline powder should contain the raw materials listed below for the best result. (The quantities cited may vary from product to product, but these are the amounts I recommend as a daily dosage.)

660 mg of tricalcium phosphate

190 mg of magnesium phosphate

90 mg of magnesium citrate

280 mg of potassium hydrogencarbonate

190 mg of potassium citrate

80 mg of calcium citrate

Many of the above substances are frequently taken individually. For example, calcium is recommended throughout the world to treat osteoporosis, and magnesium is often taken to counteract muscle cramps and stress. However, alkaline powder includes these most important mineral substances and others in balanced quantities.

The base powder may also contain other ingredients, such as selenium and zinc. Both selenium and zinc support the immune system and protect against free radicals. Also, to provide the powder with volume, "fillers" such as mannitol, a substance that cleanses the intestines and provides roughage, are often added.

As mentioned earlier, alkaline powder differs from the usually available over-the-counter antacids, which mainly protect the stomach lining or neutralize the gastric acid. They only have an effect on the stomach, while the substances of alkaline powder are absorbed in the intestines and have an effect on the entire body.

CONCLUSION

Making basic but essential lifestyle changes is critical to preventing and combating acidosis. The steps involved—proper nutrition, drinking plenty of water, regular moderate exercise, avoiding addictive substances and stress—may seem like common sense, but most of us have to make conscious adjustments to our current lifestyles to truly follow them. Use the guidelines given above to move in a healthy direction, and give yourself time to achieve them. Supplementation with alkaline powder to assist in acid reduction is a step that is new for many of us, and you may have a number of questions about it. The next chapter explains this process in more detail.

CHAPTER 5

Alkaline Powder and Deacidification Q&As

Now that you've reached this part of the book, you may be wondering exactly how to go about including alkaline powder in your detoxification plan, and you may have some questions remaining about deacidification in general. This chapter provides more detail, explaining how alkaline powder can assist the body in combating acidosis by answering questions people frequently ask about this process.

Q. *Why isn't a diet high in alkaline foods sufficient to win the battle against acidosis?*

A. As mentioned earlier, evaluating foods for their effects on the pH balance is imprecise because it relies on many factors, including whether an individual's metabolism tends toward the acid-forming or the alkali-forming range. Apart from nutrition, which certainly is an important factor, your entire lifestyle will be responsible for your metabolic tendencies. Moreover, based on experience, people can only comply with a so-called alkaline diet for a short time because it is too limiting. Simply eating only alkaline-forming foods cannot combat the acid buildup in someone whose body is excessively acidic. In other words, a glass of water cannot extinguish a burning house. It is more important to eliminate or reduce acid-forming foods and/or to eat them earlier in the day than it is to eat primarily alkaline foods. Even small amounts of acid-forming foods need to be neutralized, and alkaline foods cannot do this alone. That's why regular intake of alkaline powder is so important to a healthy acid/alkaline balance. When a person has a balanced acid/alkaline environment based on his or her positive lifestyle choices, chronic acidosis should not develop at an early age. However, at an older age, when the organs become limited in their function, the body should be supported in its fight against acidosis with alkaline powder.

Q. *How much water is necessary during deacidification?*

A. The medical rule reads as follows: The quantity of pure water consumed in liters per day should be skin surface in square meters times two. The skin surface of an average person varies between 1.5 and 2 square meters. Therefore, the average demand in liquid is between 3 and 4 liters (150–200 ounces) per day. (Salted and acid-containing beverages, such as fruit juice, alcohol, and coffee, must be *deducted* from this amount and extra water must be consumed to make up the difference.) This may sound like a lot of water, but this amount will feel natural as soon as you've reestablished a natural thirst sensation by drinking more water more often.

Q. *What's the best type of water for deacidification?*

A. High-quality natural water is best if available. Find out the source of your drinking water. If, after some investigation, you find that it is not good-quality water, purchase still mineral water. Mineral water will assist deacidification if it fulfills the following requirements:

• It must be non-carbonated.

- It should have a pH value above 7.4.

- It should be low in sodium. (Mineral water that is completely free of sodium is virtually nonexistent.)

Q. *Is it okay to drink carbonated beverages during deacidification?*

A. Avoid carbonated drinks, not only because they are highly acid forming, but also because they release gases in the intestines. Don't limit the avoidance of carbonated beverages to a specific period of deacidification; eliminate them from your diet completely and permanently.

Q. *Can herbal teas assist in the deacidification process?*

A. A number of herbal teas can assist with deacidification because they stimulate the kidneys to eliminate sodium chloride. Sodium chloride (common salt) stored in the body encourages acidosis, through fluid retention and associated weight gain. Both stinging nettle tea and dandelion tea are useful for this purpose. Refer to literature on herbal medicines to help you find other herbs that also have this beneficial effect. The amount of water in your herbal teas can be counted toward your daily intake of water.

Q. *Does the pH value of alkaline powder matter?*

A. The pH value of alkaline powder depends on the liquid in which it is dissolved. For example, alkaline powder dissolved in vinegar has a lower pH value than alkaline powder dissolved in milk. It is best to dissolve alkaline powder in pure high-quality water. The alkalinity of the powder is not the decisive factor in its efficiency.

What matters is the quality of the substances in the powder, and whether the chemical composition of the ingredients is well designed and tested.

The significant advantage of alkaline powder is in offering the body high-quality substances that stimulate it to release acid salts as well as toxins such as lead, cadmium, and mercury. Therefore, the decisive criterion of the value of an alkaline powder is this exchange action, rather than pH value. This principle applies whenever the exchange is to the advantage of the organism.

Q. *For how long should alkaline powder be taken?*

A. Many people want to know how long they should deacidify: Days, weeks, months, years? The answer lies in the fact that acid is a constant danger. For that reason, it is a good idea to take 1 heaping teaspoon of alkaline powder dissolved in a glass of water on a daily basis for the maintenance of good health. Think of it this way: Do we never have to eat again once we are full? We will always become hungry again, and in the same way, we remain exposed to the danger of acidosis.

In the case of rheumatic diseases, it may take several months before the enormous acid deposits are released from the tissues, joints, and muscles. Higher doses (two to three teaspoons daily) are needed during that time.

The amount needed on a particular day depends on person's discipline. On a day when healthy habits are maintained, a person will need less alkaline powder to feel good. If you are feeling out of sorts and have partaken in some of the unhealthy habits mentioned throughout this book, go ahead and take a teaspoon of alkaline powder to regain your well-being.

Q. *Is it possible to take too much alkaline powder?*

A. It's virtually impossible to experience side effects from the recommended doses of alkaline powder. A maximum daily dosage is five teaspoons daily, but this depends on body weight and the degree of acidosis, as well as on the state of health, lifestyle, health consciousness, and diet. The more unhealthy a person's lifestyle, the more alkaline powder he or she will require for deacidification.

A large intake of alkaline powder will have a purgative effect and might result in loose stools or diarrhea. This effect may be desirable for deacidification and intestinal cleansing, but it should only be done under a doctor's supervision. Do not take more than the maximum daily dosage unless instructed to do so by a qualified health practitioner. It is advisable to stay at home during such treatment as the intestinal-cleansing process could start suddenly and unexpectedly.

Q. *Can other supplements be taken with alkaline powder?*

A. Although alkaline powder may satisfy the daily requirements of some minerals, the main reason for taking alkaline powder is deacidification. Therefore, don't look to alkaline powder to fulfill your daily nutrient requirements. It is not advisable to take all-in-one alkaline powders—that is, powders that contain a blend of vitamins and minerals—as various unwanted reactions between nutrients are possible.

Depending on an individual's nutrient status and dietary habits, it may be advisable to take additional supplements containing trace elements and other minerals, including zinc, copper, manganese, iron, and calcium. And while it's best to get your vitamins from natural, high-quality foods, this is not always possible. Therefore, it's a good idea to take vitamin supplements on a daily basis. However, do not take any of these supplements simultaneously with alkaline powder since they may interfere with the absorption of its ingredients or cause chemical reactions. It is best to wait fifteen minutes to an hour after taking alkaline powder to take your other supplements.

After learning all you have about the acid danger, you may be worried that vitamins such as ascorbic acid and folic acid will have a damaging effect on the body. Rest assured; as far as this is concerned, the positive effects of vitamins far outweigh their acid loading. A standard dosage of these vitamins will not cause harm.

Q. *Can alkaline powder be taken with other natural remedies?*

A. Natural health practitioners and other health professionals report that certain natural remedies only become fully effective after a person has undergone deacidification. Most natural remedies agree with alkaline powder and do not hinder one another in their effects but often complement one another. In other words, in many of these naturopathic treatments, the effectiveness is actually increased by alkaline powder, as the acidosis is at least a cofactor in the development of disease. Alkaline powder increases the effectiveness of the following naturopathic treatments:

- **Ayurveda**—the ancient traditional healing system of India, which provides guidance for food intake and lifestyle habits.

- **Essential oil therapy**—the use of plant-derived

essential oils massaged into the skin for therapeutic results in body, mind, and soul.

- **Homeopathic remedies**—a medical practice based on the principles of similarity.

- **Orthomolecular preparations**—high-dose vitamin and mineral therapy.

Q. *Will alkaline powder interact with certain medications?*

A. It is recommended in principle that no medication be taken along with alkaline powder. In particular, antirheumatic medication, cortisone, and antibiotics may negatively influence the powder's effectiveness when taken at the same time. These medications are known acid producers, so although you must counteract their effects with alkaline powder, you cannot do so by taking the medication and powder simultaneously. Wait at least fifteen minutes after taking your medication to take alkaline powder.

Q. *Is it okay to take antacids and alkaline powder at the same time?*

A. Antacids are medicines that buffer gastric acid and protect the stomach lining. Their effective mechanism is different from that of alkaline powder. These medicines are severely alkaline in the stomach, but hardly cure the acidosis in the entire body. This group may be taken simultaneously with alkaline powder.

Q. *Why is sodium-free alkaline powder preferred?*

A. The value of sodium-free food and supplements is repeatedly questioned and provides a frequent discussion point for physicians and pharmacists, since sodium cannot be placed on the same footing as sodium chloride, or common salt. Sodium (also called natrium) is an element found almost everywhere. Mostly, it is combined with various other elements and very rarely appears in pure form. It shows a high affinity to chloride and forms common salt.

So, why should sodium salts in an alkaline powder be avoided? It is common to find an absolute overload of sodium chloride in the body, whereas a sodium deficiency is very rare indeed. Our foods are preserved and flavored with common salt. We consume multiple quantities of the daily requirement of sodium. The effect of a very high salt intake in the evening becomes visible the next day: puffy eyes, thirst, and fluid retention in the legs (edema). But mainly, it is our well-being that suffers from common salt because of these and other symptoms, such as high blood pressure.

The kidneys' ability to excrete acid is blocked by common salt because natrium ions put the excretory systems of kidney cells under a lot of stress and also occupy the excretory channels in the cells, causing the body to no longer be capable of excreting sufficient acid molecules to maintain a proper acid/alkaline balance. As a result, latent acidosis develops. If there is too much sodium chloride in the body, the brain tries to create a sensation of thirst, so that you drink more water and force the kidneys to eliminate the sodium chloride. That means the kidneys are once again unavailable to eliminate acid.

In short, the typical diet already contains enough salt. Experience shows that better results can be achieved with sodium-free alkaline powder. That alone substantiates that sodium is not necessary.

Q. *Why is selenium a beneficial addition to alkaline powder?*

A. Laboratory tests at the University of Graz indicate that many people have a selenium deficiency. Food alone will not provide enough daily selenium. This justifies adding selenium to alkaline powder, as long as it is added in the proper amount. Selenium is known as an important trace element, and it is a vital ingredient of enzymes that have an antioxidant effect. It protects against oxidative stress, which destroys health and is potentially harmful to well-being. Selenium also acts as an antidote against chronic stress caused by heavy metals such as lead, cadmium, and mercury. Detoxification is one of the desirable effects of alkaline powder, so it makes sense to take a selenium-containing alkaline powder.

Note that selenium is toxic in too high a dosage. For this reason, it's best to stay away from so-called homemade alkaline powder mixtures. Selenium should be added to alkaline powder only under close supervision and control. Up to 500 mcg a day will not have toxic effects. However, the amount in alkaline powder should be well below this level.

Q. *Can alkaline powder be taken during pregnancy?*

A. Extraordinary changes take place in the body of an expectant mother. Although they are normal, these changes stress the body. If this stress is not counteracted, the body will protect the unborn child at the expense of the mother. Acidosis has an easy task at overtaking the body during the nine months in which a new human being is formed. Many women report the following acid-related discomforts during pregnancy:

- Heartburn and gastroenteritis
- Lumbago (pain in the lumbar region)
- Swollen legs
- Loose teeth
- Puffy eyes

Other acid-related diseases can occur for the first time during pregnancy, or can worsen if they already exist. Medication to relieve these symptoms is often contraindicated during pregnancy due to the possible danger to the unborn child. Many pregnant women who suffer from heartburn and gastroenteritis report that these symptoms disappear completely after taking alkaline powder. However, the powder's formulation is of utmost importance. Dr. Auer's alkaline powder has been shown to be safe during pregnancy, as none of the substances included exceed the limits recommended during pregnancy. But any supplement a pregnant woman or nursing mother is considering for her daily regimen should first be cleared by her obstetrician.

Q. *Is alkaline powder safe for children?*

A. Contrary to former assumptions that children hardly ever suffer from acidosis, the nutritional habits of modern society have unfortunately changed so drastically that even infants may suffer from excess acid. This phenomenon applies in particular to overweight children in whom the acidosis is both cause and effect.

The most common symptom of acidosis in children is the so-called navel colic (stomachaches in the area of the navel). These children frequently suffer from chronic constipation and hard stools. No pathological findings can be detected during a medical examination. Upon questioning the children and their parents, it turns out that the culprit is often a diet high in sugary drinks and sweets.

The metabolic principles of adults apply to children as well. Both sugar consumption and salt intake should be reduced in children. Children should also drink more water, but this is more easily said than done since kids prefer juices and flavored instant drinks. When your child is thirsty, offer only water at certain times to get him or her used to drinking it more often.

The dosage of alkaline powder for children is slightly lower than for adults. One heaping teaspoon contains approximately 8 grams of alkaline powder. Children weighing more than 45 pounds can take the adult dosage (1 teaspoon daily as a maintenance dose). Below this weight, 2 grams of alkaline powder per 10 pounds of body weight is recommended.

Children sometimes don't like the taste of the powder, but sugar should not be added under any circumstances. Dissolve the alkaline powder in milk, and children will then enjoy the drink. Just make sure it doesn't contain any additional sugar!

Q. *Does alkaline powder help detoxify the body of heavy metals, cortisone, and antibiotics?*

A. Heavy metals (lead, mercury, cadmium, strontium, and thallium) cause many serious health problems as they accumulate in the body over the years. They interfere with metabolism by attaching themselves to proteins and peptides (rendering them inactive), functioning as enzyme poisons in the cells by displacing important trace elements and minerals from their central binding location. Heavy metals weaken the immune system and cause damage to the kidneys and liver, and lead and cadmium impair bone metabolism by obstructing absorption of calcium.

Heavy metals such as lead, cadmium, mercury, and strontium work together with acidosis to maintain and strengthen each other. In cases of existing acidosis, heavy metals are metabolized more efficiently and eliminated with more difficulty. The heavy metals thus accumulated damage biochemical and biological functions, shifting the metabolism toward the acid range and blocking the effect of alkaline-forming complexes in the body. That causes an increased and multiplied acid-loading process.

The use of alkaline components is definitely required for the elimination of heavy metals, and because selenium is an efficient detoxifier for heavy metals, it should be a component of this process. The detoxification process can take several months in the case of heavy metal contact, such as high air pollution over many years (exhaust fumes from vehicles), amalgam dental fillings, and so on. In such cases, a strong deacidification routine is required, consisting of one to two weeks using three to four heaping teaspoons of alkaline powder daily, followed by a maintenance dosage of one teaspoon daily. Depending on the case, the follow-up dosage may, at times, be increased to three to four teaspoons daily. The same process applies for patients being treated with cortisone and antibiotics. Cortisone and antibiotics often have side effects when they are taken for a long period of time. Alkaline powder will support the body by accelerating their excretions.

Q. *Why can my acidosis symptoms get worse when I start deacidification?*

A. Many patients report a worsening of their symptoms after beginning a deacidification treatment. This applies mainly in cases in which latent acidosis is quite severe and has existed for many years.

   The explanation for this phenomenon is clear. The alkaline powder releases the acids' salt deposits from organs and tissues. Initially the kidneys cannot sufficiently excrete the acids because there is not enough water available to do so. Therefore, symptoms may worsen when the treatment commences.

   Some newly released acids that cannot be flushed out immediately can deposit themselves in the loose tissue around the eyes (resulting in puffy eyes) or in the legs (resulting in edema). This is not a side effect of alkaline powder but a sign of massive acidosis. To avoid these symptoms, particularly in the beginning, it is vitally important to drink more water than you normally would (about 64–80 ounces) when you take alkaline powder. Your symptoms will not get worse despite your having severe acidosis if you do that.

Q. *When should alkaline powder be taken?*

A. Do not take alkaline powder immediately after meals as it can neutralize gastric acid, which is necessary for proper digestion. Also, gastric acid can prevent the high-quality alkaline powder components from having their full impact.

In a deacidification treatment, the powder should be taken with sufficient water approximately fifteen to twenty minutes after a meal, three times a day. The powder can also be taken independent of mealtimes. The maintenance dosage of 1 teaspoon daily should also be taken fifteen to twenty minutes after a meal.

If you want to lose weight, take the powder with lots of water fifteen minutes *before* a meal, as it will have you feel satiated sooner. You can also overcome ravenous hunger attacks with alkaline powder. If you feel hungry between meals, take the powder instead of snacking.

Sportsmen and high-performance athletes should take alkaline substances with plenty of water preferably before, as well as during and after physical activity. This causes a reduced formation of lactic acid in the muscles, and lactic acid tolerance is increased.

CONCLUSION

Alkaline powder supplementation is an excellent means for achieving overall health by fighting the effects of acidosis in the body. A quality alkaline powder should contain selenium, because they work synergistically as a particularly effective means for dealing with the stresses of long-term exposure to heavy metals, which is a cause of many serious diseases and illnesses. Alkaline powder is safe for everyone, including children and pregnant women. It is important to take a good quality powder containing the right balance of ingredients and follow proper dosage according to your particular health condition, and consume plenty of water to avoid any of the adverse effects you could experience from the initial acid elimination. These simple steps will make alkaline powder an essential and beneficial addition to your daily routine.

Conclusion

Whether young or old, achieving and maintaining good health is our most basic goal because our quality of life is influenced more by our health than by any other single factor. Our bodies are complex mechanisms affected by every aspect of our environment: the air we breathe, the food and drink we consume, and the lifestyle we follow. Scientific research continues to give us a better understanding of the human body, the illnesses that can assault it, and how we can fight to maintain and improve our health. What we have learned has shown us that we have a great deal of control over our long-term health and well-being. We can fight against the primary causes of much of the illness we experience, which often is due to an imbalance in our body's acid/alkaline levels and resulting acute or latent acidosis. Acidosis not only affects metabolism and weight, but ultimately causes almost serious disease, from diabetes, gout, and rheumatism to heart attacks and strokes.

New medical knowledge concerning the acid/alkaline balance is of great importance in your lifestyle, but knowledge alone is not enough to confront acidosis. Fighting acidosis is a critical step in maintaining or regaining your health, and you must take an active role in this battle. The acid danger waits for its chance. You have to fight against damaging acids deliberately and actively, and this requires discipline. We all are aware that making wise choices in our diet, drinking enough pure water, maintaining healthy activity levels, and keeping a positive attitude should be part of our everyday lifestyle, but a new and critical step is adding a good quality alkaline pow-der to our daily supplement routine. Many an illness can be stopped in its initial stage with this simple change. This book can help you follow proper alkaline supplementation proce-dures, and can be your most effective weapon in your fight to eliminate acidosis. Your body will thank you with lifelong activity and well-being.

References

Avenell A. et al. "Bone loss associated with high fibre weight reduction diet in postmenopausal women." *Eur J Clin Nutr* (1994): 48; 561–566.

Ball D. et al. "Blood and urine acid-base status of premenopausal omnivorous and vegetarian women." *Br J Nutr* (1997): 78; 683–693.

Barzel U.S. "The skeleton as an ion exchange system: implications for the role of acid-base imbalance in the genesis of osteoporosis." *J Bone Min Res* (1995): 10 (10); 1431–1436.

Barzel U.S. et al. "Excess dietary protein can adversely affect bone." *J Nutr* (1998): 128; 1051–1053.

Chan J.C. "Nutrition and acid-base metabolism." *Federation Proc* (1981): 40; 2423–2428.

England S.J. et al. "Fluctuation in alveolar CO_2 and in base excess during the menstrual cycle." *Respir Physiol* (1976): 26 (2); 157–161.

Fogelholm M. et al. "Association between weight cycling history and bone mineral density in premenopausal women." *Osteoporosis Int.* (1997): 7; 354–358.

Forster H.V. et al. "Estimation of arterial PO2, PCPO2, pH, and lactate from arterialized venous blood." *J Apply Physiol* (1972): 32; 134–137.

Frassetto L. et al. "Effect of age on blood acid-base composition in adult humans: role of age-related renal functional decline." *Am J Physiol* (1996): 271; F1114–F1122.

Frassetto L.A. et al. "Potassium bicarbonate reduces urinary nitrogen excretion in postmenopausal women." *J Clin Endocrinol Metab* (1997): 82; 254–259.

Frassetto L.A. et al. "Estimation of net endogenous noncarbonic acid production in humans from diet potassium and protein contents." *Am J Clin Nutr* (1998): 68; 576–583.

Frassetto L.A. et al. "Diet, evolution and aging." *Eur J Nutr* (2001): 40; 200–213.

Heavy R.P. et al. "Calcium and Weight: Clinical Studies." *J Am Coll Nutr* (2002): 21(2); 152S–155S.

Hu J.F. et al. "Dietary intakes and urinary excretion of calcium and acids: a cross-sectional study of women in China." *Am J Clin Nutr* (1993): 58; 398–406.

Linkswiller H.M. et al. "Protein-induced hypercalciuria." *Fedeation Proc.* (1981): 40; 2429–2433.

Lutz J. "Calcium balance and acid-base status of women as affected by increases protein intake and by sodium bicarbonate ingestion." *Am J Clin Nutr* (1984): 39; 281–288.

Lutz J. et al. "Calcium metabolism in postmenopausal and osteoporotic women consuming two levels of dietary protein." *Am J Clin Nutr* (1981): 34; 2178–2186.

Pilot C. et al. "Acid-base balance immediately after administration of an oral contraceptive." *Arch Gynakol* (1977) 28: 233(3); 221–231.

Preston R.J. et al. "Physiochemical analysis of phasic menstrual cycle effects on acid-base balance." *Am J Physiol Regulatory Integrative Comp Physiol* (2001): 280; R481–R487.

Remer T. et al. "Estimation of the renal net acid excretion by adults consuming diets containing variable amounts of protein." *Am J Clin Nutr* (1994): 59; 1356–1361.

Remer T. et al. "Dietary protein as a modulator of the renal net acid excretion capacity: Evidence that an increased protein intake improves the capability of the kidney to excrete ammonium." *Nutr Biochemistry* (1995): 6; 431–437.

Remer T. et al. "Influence of diet on acid-base balance." *Dialysis* (2000): 13; 221–226.

Remer T. et al. "Potential renal acid of foods and its influence on urine pH." *J Am Diet Assoc* (1995): 95; 791–797.

Sebastian A. et al. "Improved mineral balance and skeletal metabolism in postmenopausal women treated with potassium bicarbonate." *N Engl J Med* (1994): 330; 1776–1781.

Swenson E.R. "Metabolic acidosis." *Respir Care* (2001): 46 (4); 342–353.

Takano N. et al. "Renal contribution to acid-base regulation during the menstrual cycle." *Am J Physiol* (1983): 244(3); F320–324.

Zemel M.B. et al. "Regulation of adiposity by dietary calcium." *FASEB J* (2000): 14; 1132–1138.

Index

Printed in the USA
CPSIA information can be obtained
at www.ICGtesting.com
JSHW051957150824
68134JS00050B/95

9 781681 627885